GAIN MUSCLE MASS IN AN ORGANIC WAY

SIMPLE MUSCLE GAIN GUIDE

WILLIAMS SCOTT

DEDICATION

This book is dedicated to everyone who has found meaning in muscle building and its importance to them. Welcome to the community.

CONTENTS

INTRODUCTION

For those who are finding the best possible way to gain muscle mass in an organic way I can assure you that you are at the right place and at the end of this book you have a lot to fall back on and use to your advantage in your health life and your muscle growth in addition.

There are lots and lots of information and guide on gaining muscle, some give the best tips to help the user, but some even misguide the user and end up harmed and their body in a bad posture.

This book will give you the essential information, diets, and nutrients needed to supply the body with enough calories to build muscle mass healthily. There are many supplements and medications that will empower you to acquire muscle quickly. In any case, to keep away from an engineered approach, take a stab at utilizing a program of activity and natural dietary changes. By focusing on acquiring muscle naturally, you will permit your body to yield quick, amazing outcomes typically.

With regard to body enhancements, muscle building is often a first concern. Added bulk will expand the meaning of your muscles, further develop your lean weight, and add mass and size to your casing in the appropriate spots. Muscle growth takes time, determination, and a drawn-out obligation to the cycle. While acquiring a lot of muscle might appear to be overwhelming, with legitimate preparation programs and sufficient utilization of specific food sources, serious muscle building is feasible for a great many people.

Individuals frequently need to acquire muscle to put their best self forward, yet fabricating muscle has many advantages past the tasteful. With more muscle, you can be more dynamic without feeling pain the following day, make more upheld joints for more prominent adaptability, and lessen your gamble of specific infections.
To figure out how to acquire muscle rapidly and normally, you've come to the perfect locations, yet there are no enchanted responses.

WHAT IS MUSCLE MASS?

One reason I joined boxing classes quite a while back was that I trusted that preparing consistently would give me a Muhammed Ali body, and it didn't, obviously.

I missed the mark on the principle of figuring out how building muscles functions. close contact boxing gave me the important abilities for self-protection and worked on my perseverance, yet it didn't make me a John Cena lookalike.

What I just later acknowledged is that your muscles possibly develop themselves on a microscopical level as needs are. Furthermore, you, as a plainly visible human, can cultivate that need in your muscles.

To acquire muscle, you need to prepare on a particular rep range and on a particular recurrence.

IMPORTANCE OF GAINING MUSCLE MASS

Whether you lift weights or do exercises, preparing to expand your bulk, strength, and perseverance is the foundation of any workout schedule. The medical advantages of being strong incorporate quicker digestion, decreased injury risk, and further developed capacity to perform everyday tasks.

Muscles are frequently portrayed as the "motor" of your muscle-to-fat ratio and calorie-copying component. Expanded bulk can prompt less muscle-to-fat ratio, a more grounded insusceptible framework, further developed energy levels, and decreased pressure.

As we age, we experience a characteristic loss of muscle known as sarcopenia. Not in the least does this affect our typical physical processes like strolling, standing, and lifting objects, it additionally makes individuals more powerless against persistent illness. It's feasible to battle the regular rotting of bulk through strength preparation.

Another normal ailment individuals experience as they age is the debilitating of bones. At the point when bones rot, they become weak and more delicate, which expands your gamble of a crack or break. In outrageous instances of osteoporosis, something as minor as a sniffle or little knock can cause a crack. Lifting loads can assist with expanding bone thickness and bone strength.

Helps bring down your resting pulse. Testing yourself with significant burden preparation is believed to be particularly important since heavier loads cause more effort on the cardiovascular framework.

Battling coronary illness and type 2 diabetes. There is proof to propose that strength preparation can work on the body's resilience to glucose as well as insulin awareness. Both are significant variables in the body's guideline of glucose levels.

It also helps in directing muscle-to-fat ratio levels. Raised degrees of muscle-to-fat ratio can prompt serious negative circumstances, from coronary illness to hypertension to unnecessary wear on joints and bones.

Past these entire body physiological advantages of bulk, the cycle by which we assemble muscle - opposition work out - is additionally connected with upgrades in psychological well-being, which thusly influences our general personal satisfaction.

As may be obvious, fabricating and keeping up with bulk is quite possibly the main thing you can accomplish for your well-being.

HEALTHY VS UNHEALTHY MUSCLE GAIN

To gain muscles in any case, you need to put your body under pressure. Preparing itself isn't completely good for you. You're losing valuable body liquids in the exercise center, exhausting your energy assets, and making miniature tears in your muscles. It's just when your body feels awkward that you fabricate muscles in any case.

Getting more fit is likewise a distressing circumstance for your body for the time being. You're taking in less energy than your body wants, which powers your body to rebuild your life form such that needs less energy. In a non-logical term: Your body begins consuming fat on the off chance that you eat less calories.

Keep in mind, healthy is dependably relative. Driving a liquor fiend to quit drinking might hurt them radically temporarily, with respect to pressure chemicals, however in the drawn out it very well may be an extraordinary choice when we think about the other option.

In the feeling of figuring out how to acquire muscle, outrageous muscle gain may be destructive, yet on the off chance that the option is weight, it tends to be viewed as solid, as it builds the future for the singular more than being obese.

What makes muscle gain healthy is the recuperation stage. The zenith of sound muscle gain is doing it on a plant-based diet, with a lot of rest and a pressure-lessening individual life. Likewise, without the assistance of anabolic steroids, obviously.

IS THERE ANY RISK TO INCREMENT MUSCLE MASS?

Building causes gigantic stress on bone-muscle connectors. Adding an abundance of weight will drive an unfortunate burden on tendons and ligaments. It's vital to comprehend that these urgent connectors don't develop, as body creation becomes controlled during the building system.

Lifting too much weight or moving in an unusual manner in an effort to build muscles **could result in a muscle tear as well as damage to ligaments and tendons as well as the surrounding soft tissue**.

A person who is attempting to get in shape and construct bulk at the same time may at first put on weight. This condition is transitory. While initially beginning your eating routine and strength-preparing program, your expansion in bulk might dominate your deficiency of fat.

Utilizing lighter loads and doing more redundancies can limit the building impact causing your weight gain or level. Talking with a wellness mentor gives you customized and proficient assistance to invalidate this drawback of building muscle mass.

Watch your eating routine to assist with dealing with the negatives of working out, for example, weight gain. Center around lean protein sources and pick foods grown from the ground as your starches. Incorporate cardio practice in your gym routine daily schedule to assist with dealing with your weight, according to ExRx.net.

The Habitats for Infectious prevention and Counteraction suggests at least 150 minutes of moderate-power or 75 minutes of enthusiastic power oxygen-consuming activity each week to keep a solid weight.

Stress Breaks in Weightlifters
A pressure break presents as a small break in your bone, according to Mayo Clinic. Leaving on an exercise program too seriously and excessively fast, alongside lifting more weight than you can deal with, can cause this skeletal injury and addresses one of the impediments to building muscle mass.

Moreover, the weighty burdens and redundancies related to weight training and strength preparation can cause pressure cracks. To stay away from pressure breaks while building bulk, a lady who is flabby should expand the power of her exercises steadily.

HEALTHY DIETS TO GAIN MUSCLE MASS

Probably, your body can add around 227 (a portion of a pound) of bulk consistently. Thusly, in the event that you consume a ton of extra calories while attempting to construct muscle, you are probably going to acquire an overabundance of fat too. A day-to-day increment of 250 to 500 calories is suggested.

Attempt to remain on the lower end of the reach assuming you gain fat effectively, and hold back nothing end of the reach in the event that you find it hard to put on weight generally. Tracking down the perfect proportion of additional calories to fabricate muscle and remain slender will take some experimentation.

Additionally, research recommends that eating lean protein 15 to 20 minutes prior to, during, and in the span of one hour of working out may assist with expanding bulk. While you are probably not going to eat steaks or chicken bosoms at the exercise center, a protein drink or enhancement might be gainful previously, during, or after exercises.

However, it's not about protein. To fabricate muscle, lose fat, and get more grounded, a solid, adjusted diet ought to give you numerous dinners that meet your caloric uses and give you sustenance. The following are eight extraordinary thoughts to assist you with building bulk.

1. Breakfast will assist with building muscle

You'll require a quick explosion of energy and breakfast will assist with giving you this. It'll likewise assist you with remaining full until your next feast or tidbit. It likewise starts the precedent: you will generally eat better in the event that your day begins with areas of strength for a sound breakfast. Your smartest choices assuming you're attempting to construct bulk are omelets, smoothies, and curds.

2. Eat Like clockwork

Eating the proper thing brilliantly is essential for assisting you with helping your bulk. The least demanding way is to have your morning meal, lunch, and supper to no one's surprise, scattered with feasts post-exercise, pre-bed, and with two in the middle between.

By keeping your food consumption up, it will mean you will not be as ravenous, on the grounds that eating more modest feasts all the more frequently versus a couple of large dinners will diminish your stomach size. You'll feel full more rapidly and your midriff will manage, while you'll likewise have fewer desires.

Not eating for extensive stretches can make you over-eat at the following feast or garnish yourself up with unfortunate snacks from the candy machine. So to stop any desires, eat at fixed times consistently and your body will get eager at those decent times.

3. Protein with every feast assists lift with muscling mass

You want protein to construct and keep up with bulk. To accomplish this, you ought to be hoping to eat no less than 1g per 454g of body weight. That is 200g/day assuming you weigh 91kg.

The most straightforward method for getting this sum is to eat an entire protein source with every dinner. These include:

- Red meat. Meat, pork, sheep, and so forth.
- Poultry. Chicken, turkey, duck, and so on.
- Fish. Fish, salmon, sardines, mackerel, and so on.
- Eggs. Try not to trust the cholesterol legends. Eat the yolk.
- Dairy. Milk, cheddar, curds, quark, yogurt, and so forth.
- Whey. Excessive however extraordinary for simple post-exercise shakes.
- Veggie lover choices like lentils, tofu, seeds, and nuts.

4. Eat Leafy foods with every dinner
A large portion of them (not all) are low calorie: you can eat your stomach full without acquiring fat or weight. Leafy foods are likewise brimming with nutrients, minerals, cell reinforcements and fiber which helps to process, yet be mindful so as to check the sugar content of certain natural products.

5. Eat carbs solely after your exercise
While you want carbs for energy, the vast majority eat an overabundance. Limit your sugar admission to after your exercise just and you'll begin constructing a lot of fit bulk.

Eat leafy foods with all feasts. These contain not many carbs contrasted with entire grains except for corn, carrots, and raisins.
Another Carbs Post Exercise As it were. This is rice, pasta, bread, potatoes, quinoa, oats, and so forth. Stay away from white carbs and eat entire grains where conceivable.

6. Practice good eating habits fat to assist with building muscle mass
Practicing good eating habits fats works on fat misfortune and by and large well-being as they digest gradually. Thusly, this will assist you with building fit bulk.

Ensure you balance your fat admission, practice good eating habits and fats with each dinner and stay away from counterfeit trans-fats and margarine. These are monounsaturated and polyunsaturated fats that you'll track down in specific food varieties. These include:

Vegetable oils, including olive and sunflower.
Nuts and seeds.
Slick fish like mackerel and salmon.

7. Drinking water assists you with building muscle mass
Strength preparation causes water misfortune through perspiring which can disable muscle recuperation. Subsequently, in the event that you don't supplant that water, all the strength preparing on the planet won't assist you with expanding your bulk. Drinking a lot of water forestalls lack hydration as well as craving since an unfilled stomach can make you believe you're ravenous.

8. Eat entire food sources 90% of the time
To truly obtain the outcomes you need and to support your bulk essentially, 90% of your food admission ought to comprise entire food sources. Attempt and stay away from handled food sources however much as could reasonably be expected.

Entire food varieties. These are natural and raw (or minimal refined) food varieties that come as close as conceivable to their regular state. Instances of these are new meat, fish, poultry, eggs, vegetables, beats, organic products, rice, oats, quinoa, and so forth.

Handled food sources for the most part contain added sugars, trans-fats, nitrates, corn syrup, sodium, and more synthetic substances. Models incorporate bagels, organic product bars, oats, pizza, treats, wieners, frozen dinners, supplements

Obviously, it's not just about getting your eating regimen right with regard to building bulk. You really want to get your exercises right, as well. Investing sufficient energy in the rec center, and doing the right activities is totally fundamental to accomplishing the additions you're searching for.

IMPORTANCE OF CONSISTENCY IN DIET FOR MUSCLE GAIN

Consistency is the key to advance in muscle gain. Anything that we complete throughout everyday life, we will absolutely not make the progress we need except if we work at it.

According to Ryan Mitchell Rios and Mark Atalla, consistency in your efforts leads to self-discipline, teaches you self-control, improves your overall personality, and builds momentum. "When you are consistent, you have a sense of accountability and direction that translates to progress," asserts the two entrepreneurs,

Consistency is the way to advance in muscle building. Anything we complete throughout everyday life, we will surely not make the progress we need except if we work at it all the time reliably. Exactly the same pick your exercise programs. You can have the absolute best educator on the planet, as well as the best eating regimen intended to follow, yet on the off chance that you don't stay with it predictably, you will without a doubt end up wasting your time. This can be very baffling for an individual that is attempting to hit a specific objective.

Tips to Consistency

I feel there are three essential components in any exercise program to build lean strong tissue and shed unfortunate muscle-to-fat ratio. These parts are opposition preparation, cardio workout, and appropriate sustenance. Every one of the three is comparatively fundamental in accomplishing your goals in wellness.

In the event that one isn't performed predictably, the different other two will without a doubt persevere and thus will surely your movement. Try not to acquire me wrong; to expect we can be ideal always will unquestionably be getting ourselves in a position for disappointment. Our objective should be to follow our projects the best we can ordinary more often than not. The more extended the second you stay with something, the greatly improved you will turn out to be grinding away. We should survey a few techniques we can keep on being extra steady with our exercise programs.

1. Strength Training

Contingent on your objectives, you ought to play out some opposition preparing with loads somewhere in the range of 3-6 times every week. The meaning of obstruction preparation is that it will unquestionably help support your lean, tone, and weight, subsequently giving a greatly improved shape to the body and furthermore expanding your fundamental metabolic rate. Muscle resembles a 24-hour radiator, so we need to ensure we keep or even improve our fit bulk to keep up with the digestion developing.

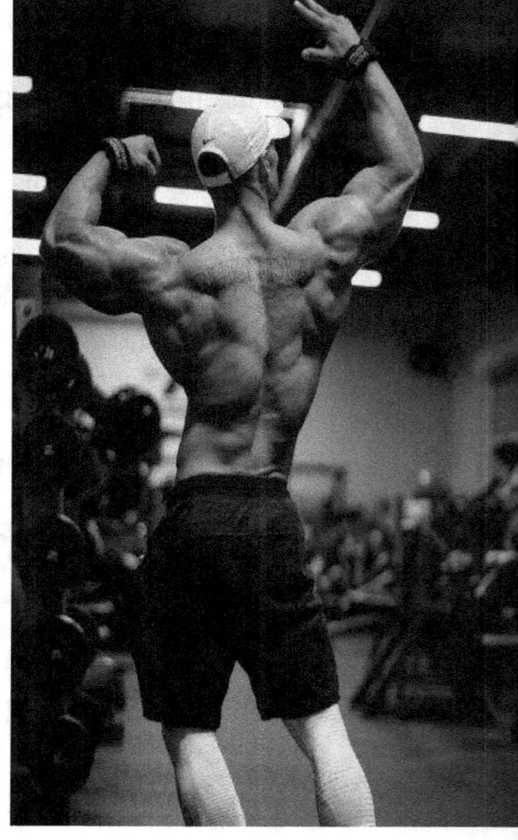

To help you to remain faithful; I would find an exercise sidekick or work with the assistance of a certified individual coach. As such, you have a responsible accomplice. It is bound to go to the exercise center assuming I realize an individual is sitting tight for you that you are liable for. Moreover having a preparation accomplice or coach will surely keep you extra focused and propelled all through your exercises as well as will keep up with you from getting exhausted from the standard, worn-out everyday practice.

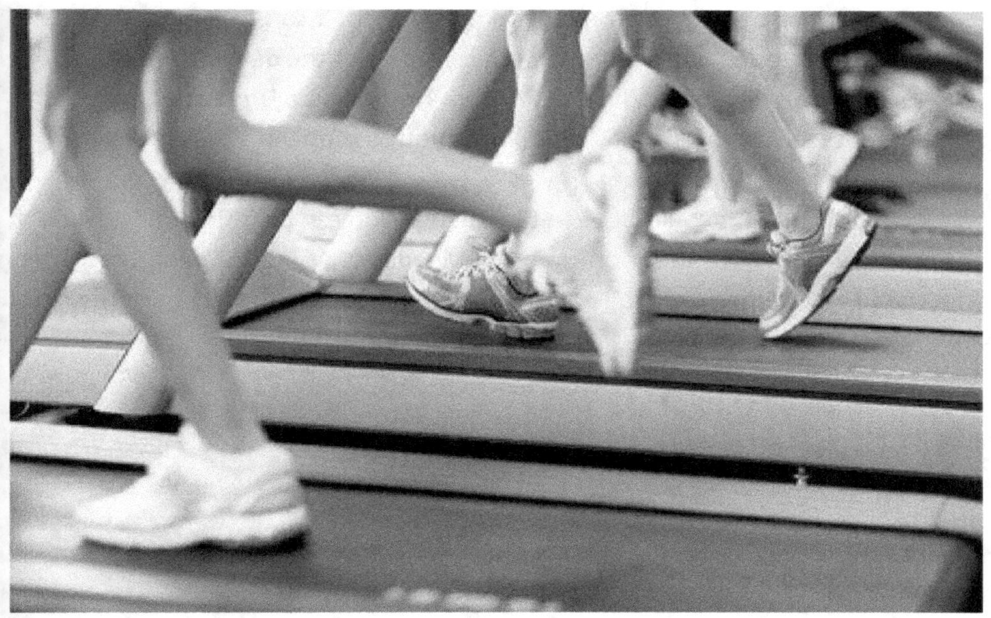

The cardiovascular assignment is vital for keeping the digestion thundering and furthermore helps you to consume a few extra calories that will without a doubt bring about fat misfortune. The fundamental variable I decide to do a lot of cardio is that it permits me to eat significantly more food nevertheless making the fat misfortune results I'm searching for. Certain individuals that rely upon diet alone to lose fat, for the most part, find themselves decreasing weight yet moreover a ton of solid tissue. Keeping some additional food in the eating routine, yet utilizing cardio to shed much more calories will without a doubt end up in the maintenance of slender muscle while shedding the fat.

I would positively prompt doing your cardio absolutely first thing, thirty minutes also, prior to morning dinner. As such, it runs out of the way, and it will upgrade your energy for a decent part of the day to consent to. It is somewhat difficult at first, but following seven days, you will without a doubt feel improved, and this will spur you to keep up.

Assuming there could be no alternate way you can do it first thing, I would surely do it just after you train with loads or around evening time after your last dinner. Carry a headset with your favored tunes to assist the time going a lot quicker.

3. Nutrition

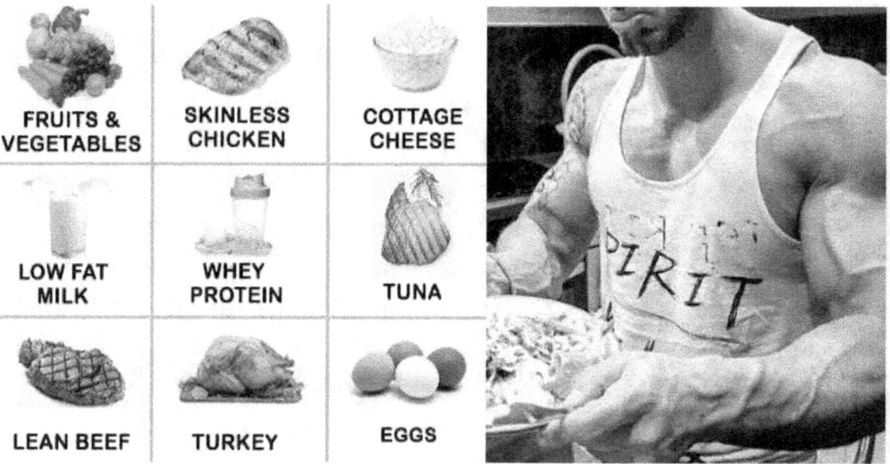

This is where I find that the most conspicuous fluctuation relies on most of the individuals. Some are really great for 2-3 days, after that blow it for 2 days, etc.

This endless loop will bring about frustration. As opposed to consenting to an outrageous eating routine technique, I rather you stick to a humble sustenance plan as well as one you believe you can follow consistently for a ton of the time. Find a technique that is loaded up with the solid and adjusted food varieties you like.

NO this doesn't recommend frozen yogurt, once in that frame of mind while, you can charm as well as appreciate it. Modest quantities are the mystery.

On the off chance that you screw up as well as appreciate 1 or 2 of your feasts, the day isn't annihilated, begin back to your eating routine arrangement for your next dinner following.

Solace is an enormous viewpoint that influences the consistency of eating the best food varieties. I propose you get in the daily schedule of setting up your feasts ahead of time. This will eliminate the purpose behind visiting a comfort food place since you don't have anything to eat. It will positively dispose of the justification behind missing a genuinely necessary dish.

I would without a doubt invest some energy and money in setting up the food myself. The most striking component of setting up your dishes is that you perceive precisely exact thing you are eating. This way you have unlimited oversight of the food you eat.

To speed up the metabolic rate and furthermore to help recover from your preparation, attempt to consume 5-6 little dinners day to day. It requires something like 2 weeks of a reliable eating project to begin helping your metabolic interaction as well as obtain results with respect to incline strong tissue gain and furthermore weight reduction. Supplement business today simplified it to strike your dishes in general.

You can procure a protein powder, a dish substitute bundle, solid protein drinks in a can currently blended, and sound protein bars. By and by, these guides eliminate any legitimization for not acquiring the legitimate nourishment your body needs.

I would in any case rather you eat entire food sources, yet something is obviously better than literally nothing at all.

Building bulk and furthermore significance is difficult work and furthermore needs a right eating routine intend to make it happen. Improve your sustenance for strong tissue advancement and forestall common mistakes, like confining calories.

NUTRITION AND MUSCLE BUILDING

To make gains you must have the right nutrients in your body to develop muscle. This implies that what you eat, and how much, is fundamental in making muscle gains. Lifting and doing strength preparation without sufficient sustenance, particularly without enough protein, can really prompt the loss of muscle tissue.

While building muscle, your body needs more fuel than while it's keeping up with body synthesis. This can be a troublesome idea for certain individuals to get a handle on. They might oppose, particularly those stressed over weight gain or acquiring fat.

you have to understand that the additional calories will go into muscle improvement, not fat, for however long you are resolving in the right manner.

Precisely the number of calories an individual needs each day while working out and acquiring muscle changes. You'll have to take a close look independently to suggest calorie consumption during a muscle-building period. For the most part, adding 20 to 30 grams of added protein each day is a decent rule for a muscle-building feast plan.

Common Nourishment Mistakes When Attempting to Build Muscle

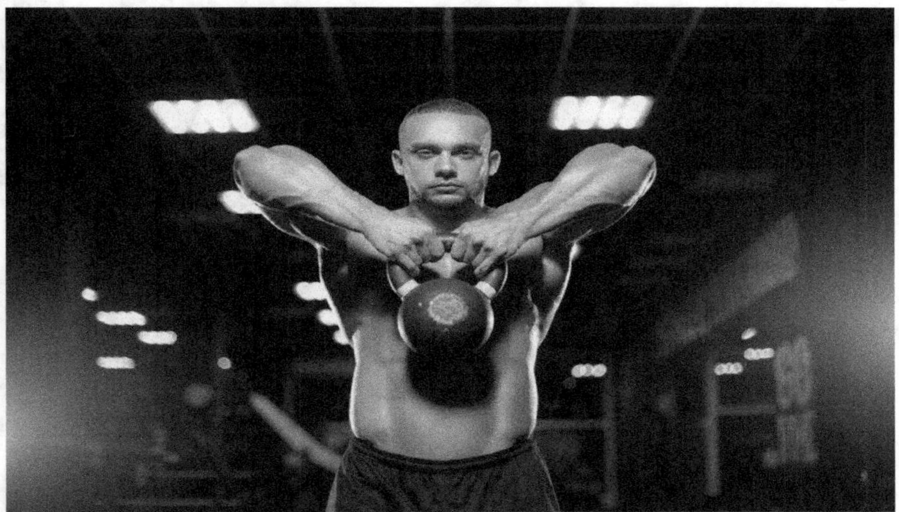

When trying to build muscle, individuals frequently make the error of restricting caloric intake from a particular sort of nutrient or restricting total calories. Make sure you satisfy every one of the nutritional requirements for muscle mass growth.

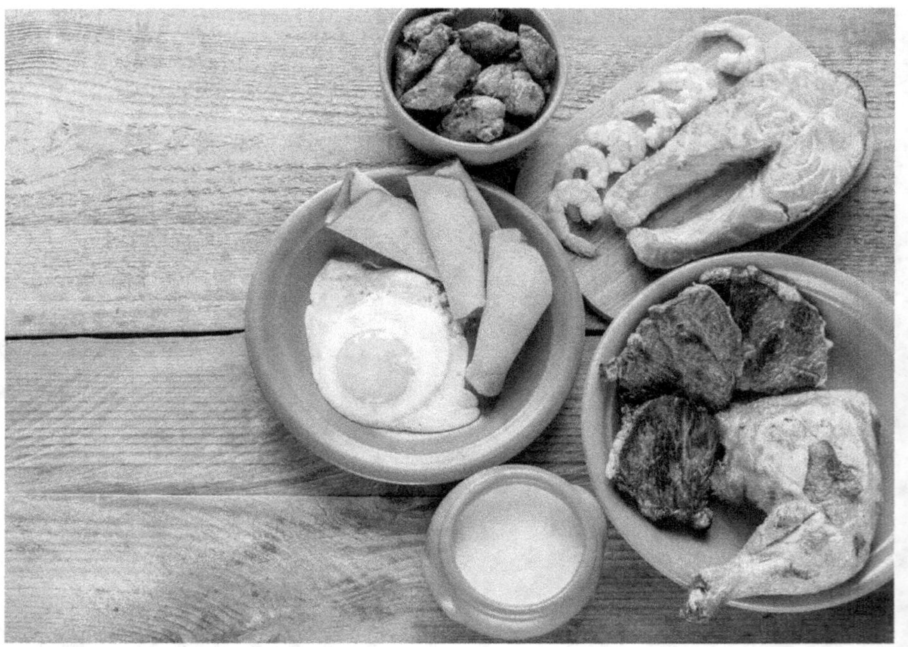

Select superior grade, high-protein sources that assist with building bulk previously and furthermore after exercises. Select genuine food over solid protein powders and even shakes, one, for example,

Eggs.
Hen and turkey bosom.
Salmon as well as fish.
Lean meats.
Soybeans and furthermore tofu.
Beans and vegetables.
Substantially more sound protein is required in your eating routine while changing to a work-out routine made to foster bulk. At the point when you are stationary, you could require 0.36 grams of protein per pound of body weight4 (or around 54 grams for a 150-pound lady and furthermore 72

grams for a 200-pound male). Assuming you are endeavoring to develop muscle, help your utilization to 0.55 to 0.77 grams of protein per pound.5.

Consume Much More Carbs.

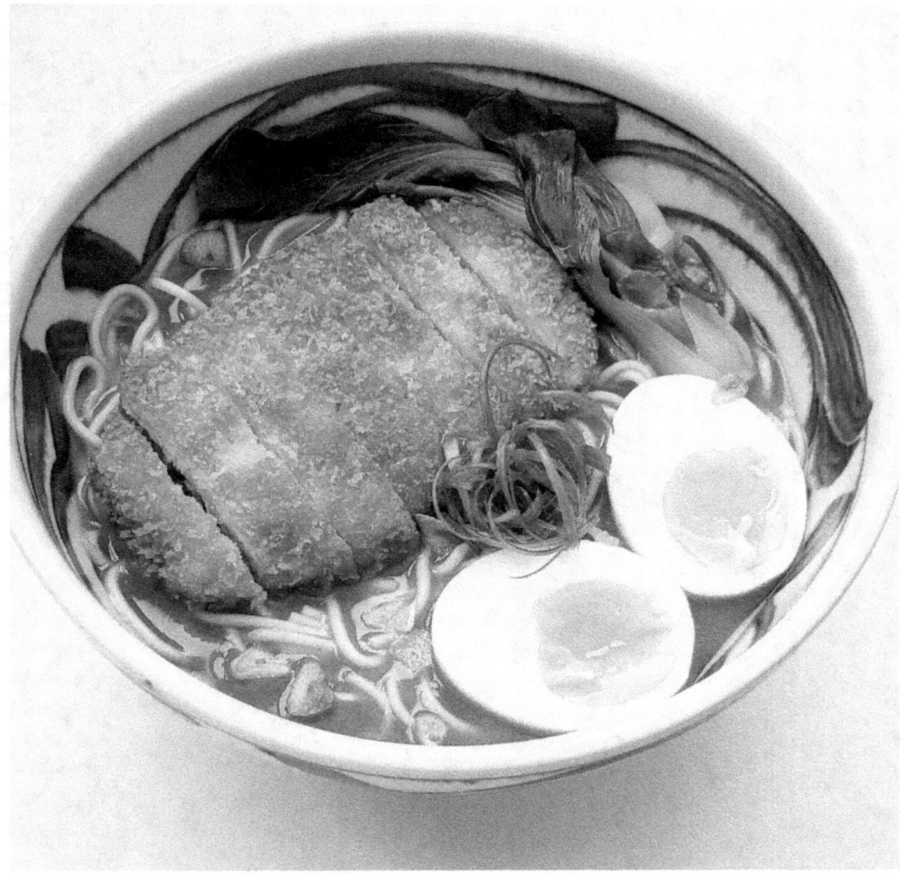

Select supplement thick sources that keep up with the glycogen stores fundamental for you to have the option to resolve longer and more effectively for example,

Sweet potatoes
Vegetables
Quinoa
Buckwheat
Root vegetables
Winter weather months squash
As liked as low-carb diets might be, they might diminish your game's execution and furthermore leave your solid tissues hurting for supplements fundamental for bulk sound protein combination.

Eat More Fats

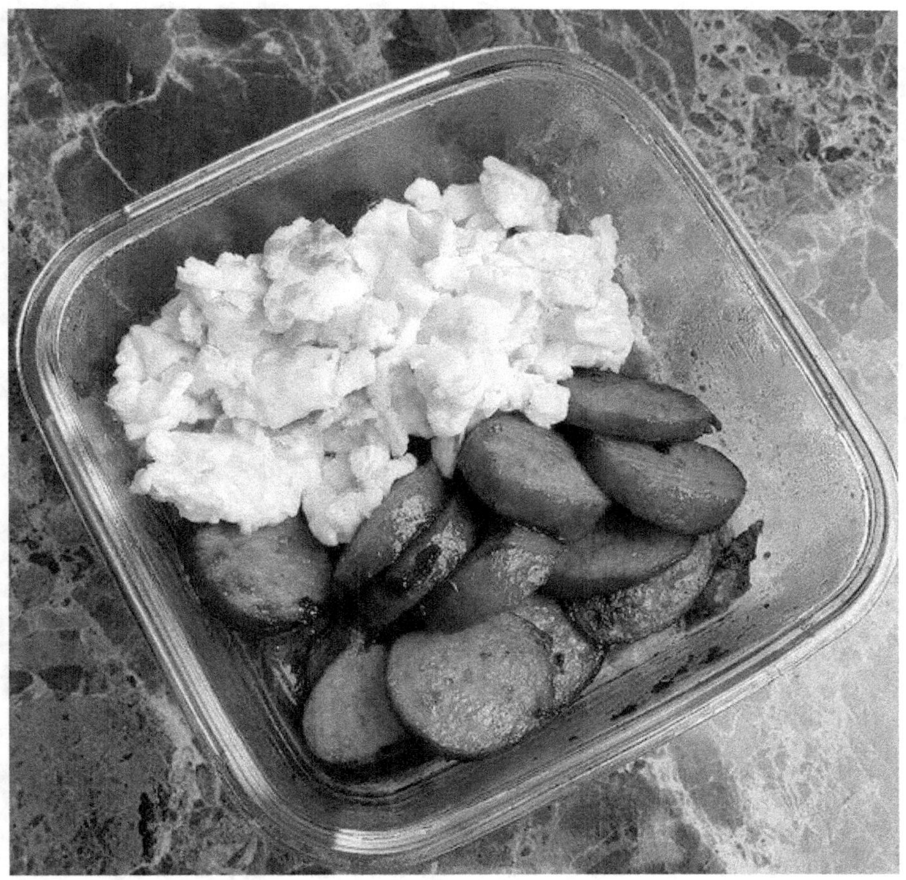

While it could assist with cutting the immersed as well as trans fats, you actually require an optimal amount of sound fats to work on metabolic rate and safeguard hormonal component. A sans fat eating regimen plan can hamper mass muscle development in a person that strongly works out. Keep fats in the vicinity of around 15% to 20 percent of your everyday caloric admission.

Sound and adjusted fats incorporate something other than olive oil. There are various different assets, both for food arrangement as well with respect to eating, comprising of:

- Avocados.
- Greek yogurt.
- Nuts as well as chia seeds.
- Olives.
- Dull delightful chocolate.
- Ghee.

Eat Significantly More, Not Substantially less.

Muscle is the gas your body will look to when your calories are diminished. At the point when you don't eat to the point of keeping up with mass muscle development, your body will go into malnourishment setting as well as increment as gone against decrease fat shops.

Assuming you are working on a mission to foster muscle, there is compelling reason need to restrict calories to at the same time lessen weight. Safeguard an even eating routine of fundamental sound proteins, carbs, as well as fats, as well as your body design will without a doubt work on after some time.

A steady routine will require a long time to create. Following a little while, it will turn out to be essential for your regular daily practice. When you strike that level, it is smooth cruising, basically "auto-pilot." Sure, in the beginning, it will positively be troublesome some of the time to set up the entirety of your feasts, hit the treadmill, as well as hit each instructional course.

You will without a doubt become accustomed to it, as well as there will without a doubt come where you won't likewise consider it since it will positively be a reliable piece of your day to day daily practice. You basically need to persuade yourself that you can make it happen and presenting individually to show up. The additional time you put in, the more certainty you will make to remain with it.

THE MUSCLE MASS ROUTINE

Might it be said that you are a middle-of-the-road or high-level learner hoping to assemble MUSCLE MASS quickly? Assuming this is the case, welcome to the program I basically call The Muscle Mass Routine.

The Muscle Mass Routine is the weight-lifting program that I prescribe most frequently to individuals hoping to construct any measure of muscle mass as quickly as could be expected.

This exercise routine is intended to work for all kinds of people, youthful and old, individuals hoping to fabricate a lot of muscle and get "enormous" or construct a modest quantity of muscle and simply get "conditioned."

Essentially, assuming that you're past the amateur stage and your essential objective is building muscle or further developing the manner in which your body thoroughly searches in basically any limit, this program is for you.

Presently we should get down to the subtleties…

The Timetable
The Muscle Mass Routine purposes an upper/lower split, which is one of the most demonstrated and well-known preparing parts ever.

One explanation the upper/lower split gets such a lot of adoration is on the grounds that it considers each muscle bunch/body part to be prepared somewhat between once every third and fifth day relying upon the particular split variety you pick (erring on those in a moment).

Furthermore, as I've recently made sense of, this exercise recurrence of about two times seven days is deductively demonstrated to turn out best for building muscle for anybody past the novice's stage.

In this way, we should investigate the 2 most normal forms of the upper/lower split…

Upper/Lower Split: multi-Day Adaptation
Monday: Chest area An Exercise
Tuesday: Lower Body An Exercise
Wednesday: off
Thursday: Chest area B Exercise
Friday: Lower Body B Exercise
Saturday: off
Sunday: off
In this multi-day variant, each muscle bunch gets prepared once every third or fourth day, which is right inside the ideal recurrence range for building Muscle Mass at the ideal rate.

While this particular layout is presumably the most widely recognized (individuals like having ends of the week off), the specific days you pick truly don't make any difference as long as a similar 2 on/1 off/2 on/2 off the design is held together.

Upper/Lower Split: multi-Day Variant
Week 1

Monday: Chest area An Exercise
Tuesday: off
Wednesday: Lower Body An Exercise
Thursday: off
Friday: Chest area B Exercise
Saturday: off
Sunday: off
Week 2

Monday: Lower Body B Exercise
Tuesday: off
Wednesday: Chest area An Exercise
Thursday: off
Friday: Lower Body An Exercise
Saturday: off
Sunday: off

In this multi-day adaptation, each muscle bunch gets prepared once every fourth or fifth day. While it is simply somewhat less continuous than the multi-day rendition, it's still impeccably inside the ideal recurrence range for building bulk at the ideal rate.

Yet again, while this layout is generally the most well-known, the specific days you pick don't make any difference whatsoever as long as a similar 1 on/1 off/1 on/1 off/1 on/2 off the design is kept in consideration.

Presently Select Your Rendition Of The Upper/Lower Split

Thus, those are the two planning choices for The Muscle Mass Routine everyday practice. You should simply pick one.

The two of them will work impeccably, so you genuinely can't turn out badly with one or the other rendition. Simply pick the one that appears to be best for you, your inclinations, and your timetable.

In the event that you really want assistance choosing, look at my more nitty gritty breakdown of the two forms here: upper/lower split.
The Exercises
Very much like most powerlifting programs worked around the upper/lower split, The Muscle Mass Routine partitions everything into 2 distinct kinds of exercises.

One will prepare your whole chest area somewhat (chest, back, shoulders, biceps, and rear arm muscles), and one will prepare your whole lower body somewhat (quads, hamstrings, calves, and abs also).

You will then do 2 (or around 2) of every exercise each week contingent upon precisely which variety of the split you choose to utilize (once more, either will be great).

Thus, we should investigate the exercises…

The Muscle Mass Routine Daily schedule: Chest area A
Seat Press
3 arrangements of 6-8 reps.
2-3 minutes rest between sets.

Columns
3 arrangements of 6-8 reps.
2-3 minutes rest between sets.

Slant Hand weight Press
3 arrangements of 8-10 reps.
1-2 minutes rest between sets.

Lat Pull-Downs
3 arrangements of 8-10 reps.
1-2 minutes rest between sets.

Horizontal Raises
2 arrangements of 10-15 reps.
brief reprieve between sets.

Rear arm muscles Pushdowns
3 arrangements of 10-12 reps.
brief reprieve between sets.
Hand weight Twists
2 arrangements of 12-15 reps.
brief reprieve between sets.

The Muscle Mass Routine Daily practice: Lower Body A
Romanian Deadlifts
3 arrangements of 6-8 reps.
2-3 minutes rest between sets.

Leg Press
3 arrangements of 10-12 reps.
1-2 minutes rest between sets.

Situated Leg Twists
3 arrangements of 8-10 reps.
1-2 minutes rest between sets.

Standing Calf Raises

4 arrangements of 6-8 reps.
1-2 minutes rest between sets.

Abs
x arrangements of 8-15 reps.
brief reprieve between sets.
The Muscle Mass Routine Daily schedule: Chest area B
Pull-Ups
3 arrangements of 6-8 reps.
2-3 minutes rest between sets.

Free weight Shoulder Press
3 arrangements of 6-8 reps.
2-3 minutes rest between sets.

Situated Link Column
3 arrangements of 8-10 reps.
1-2 minutes rest between sets.

Free weight Seat Press
3 arrangements of 8-10 reps.
1-2 minutes rest between sets.
Free weight Flyes
2 arrangements of 10-15 reps.
brief reprieve between sets.

Free weight Twists
3 arrangements of 10-12 reps.
brief reprieve between sets.

Skull Smashers
2 arrangements of 12-15 reps.
brief reprieve between sets.

The Muscle Building Gym routine Daily practice: Lower Body B
Squats
3 arrangements of 6-8 reps.
2-3 minutes rest between sets.

Divide Squats
3 arrangements of 8-10 reps.
1-2 minutes rest between sets.

Lying Leg Twists
3 arrangements of 10-12 reps.
1-2 minutes rest between sets.

Situated Calf Raises
4 arrangements of 10-15 reps.
1-2 minutes rest between sets.

Abs
x arrangements of 8-15 reps.
brief reprieve between sets.

As you can see from the exercises, every one is centered basically around the best compound activities with a perfect proportion of optional spotlight on confinement practices too.

There is additionally damn close to consummate equilibrium among the contradicting development designs, and the practices in every exercise are requested as far as generally requesting to least requesting (the specific way it ought to be).

As may be obvious, the power/rep ranges and rest spans between sets for each exercise is the precisely exact thing they ought to be for building muscle, and the volume for each muscle bunch both per exercise and each week all out is all impeccably inside the ideal volume range for halfway/high-level learners hoping to fabricate bulk.

Thus, what I'm attempting to say is, the elements as a whole and parts that turn out best for building muscle have been united entirely in one ideal exercise routine daily practice.

Exercise Request and Planning
As displayed, The Muscle Mass Routine contains 4 unique exercises. There are 2 chest area exercises (An and B) and 2 lower body exercises (An and B).

In the event that it isn't adequately clear, they are intended to be finished in a specific order whether you utilize the 3 or multi-day upper/lower split:

- Chest area A
- Lower Body A
- Chest area B
- Lower Body B

(In the event that this is as yet confounding, simply return to the upper/lower split choices I showed you before. I've spread out how you'd plan the 4 exercises throughout the span of the week utilizing either form of the split.)

Subtleties, Rules, and Explanations
Presently to address any inquiries you might have, clear up any disarray that might be available, and clarify how to make everything function as actually as could be expected.

Common rules of The Muscle Mass Routine everyday practice:

For each activity, you ought to utilize a similar weight each set. Meaning, on the off chance that it says to complete 3 arrangements of activity, you'd utilize a similar load on each of the 3 sets. For instance...
Right Way: 100lbs, 100lbs, 100lbs.
Incorrect Way: 95lbs, 100lbs, 105lbs.

At the point when you can lift a given load for how many sets and reps are endorsed for that activity, you'd then expand the load by the littlest conceivable addition the following time you do that activity. You'd then recurrent this course of movement as frequently as possible. (I'll make sense of this in significantly more detail in a moment.)
The quantity of sets recorded does exclude warm-up sets. Those are the genuine work sets as it were. Warm up on a case-by-case basis.
The request the activities are recorded in is the request they should be finished in. Try not to transform it.
You are intended to do every one of the activities recorded for every exercise. Be that as it may, on the off chance that you go over something your rec center doesn't have or something you sincerely can't do because of some prior injury (or another Truly valid justification), do the following nearest match all things considered. (I'll give a few ideas underneath.)

The split, recurrence, practice determination, recommended measure of sets, reps and rest stretches for each activity, the aggregate sum of volume... it's everything for an explanation and it is undeniably intended to remain and be done Precisely as I have composed it.

Subtleties and explanations for Chest area A:
The Chest area An exercise begins with the seat press. This is implied by a level hand-weight seat press. I suggest having a spotter if conceivable. Other than being significant for clear security reasons, not having one might make you scared of going after for an extra rep, and this could obstruct your advancement.

Up next is a line, which fundamentally implies a flat draw of some sort (significance back column workout). Essentially any kind of back column would be fine here, so pick your #1. In the event that I needed to make an idea, I could go with a chest-upheld line or some likeness thereof on the grounds that chest-upheld paddling requires no genuine lower back adjustment like a twisted-around-hand weight column would.

What's more, since you will be deadlifting the following day, this might be a useful decision for certain individuals. In any case, feel free to pick any sort of flat back column you need (chest upheld line, any Sledge Strength machine column in the event that your rec center has them, a twisted around hand weight or hand weight column, ski lift pushes, no big deal either way). However long it's a back column or some likeness thereof, it's fine. In the event that you think you'd profit from not utilizing any lower back the day preceding doing deadlifts, then, at that point, stay with something chest upheld to offer your lower back a reprieve. On the off chance that not, pick anything.

For slant squeezing, I suggest slant-free weight presses. Actually, any kind of grade press will do here. Hand weight, free weight, machine (Sledge Strength makes a grade chest press that I love). Yet, my best option proposal would be for the slope hand weight press (in which case make certain to set the seat to a 30-degree slant or somewhat less, not more).

For lat pull-downs, I suggest utilizing an underhand hold (meaning your palms will confront you) or an unbiased grasp (palms face one another… this hold is considerably less upsetting on your elbows/wrists). This is on the grounds that I will suggest an overhand hold (palms face away from you) during the Chest area B exercise. You'll see. Additionally, these are to be finished before your head… never behind the neck.

For lateral raises, you can truly do anything that parallel raise you to need. With hand weights (situated or standing, each arm in turn or both together), with links, with a sidelong raise machine in the event that your exercise center has a good one. Simply pick your #1.

For the rear arm muscles workout, I suggest link press downs utilizing essentially anything that sort of handles you like best. I for one lean toward the v-bar or rope.

For the biceps practice on this day, I suggest any kind of hand-weight twist (standing, situated, on an evangelist seat, no difference either way). Pick your number one.

Subtleties and explanations for Lower Body A:
The Lower Body An exercise starts with the Romanian deadlift. I suggest involving a twofold overhand hold rather than a blended grasp (which would be one hand north of, one hand under).

For the leg squeezes, you can do these the conventional way (the two legs simultaneously) or single leg if conceivable. Likewise, this is intended to be finished in a 45-degree leg press. On the off chance that your exercise center doesn't have one, then, at that point, utilize anything leg press they do have.

For the leg twists, a few exercise centers have at least a couple sorts of leg twist machines… situated, standing, and laying. You can truly pick anyone you need.

Next up is standing calf raises. In the event that your exercise center doesn't have a standing calf raise machine, go ahead and do calf presses in the 45-degree leg press.

For abs, do a couple of sets of anything you desire. Simply don't go too off the deep end… something like 10 minutes or somewhere in the vicinity. I love essential stuff like weighted crunches, hanging leg raises, boards, and so on.. Keep it straightforward.

Subtleties and explanations for Chest area B:

The Chest area B exercise begins with pull-ups. Utilize an overhand grasp. In the event that you can't do pull-ups, you can do lat pull-downs or some type of helped pull-up in its place (actually utilizing an overhand grasp). It's fine. In any case, you ought to make it your possible objective to have the option to do pull-ups and really pursue in the long run doing them here. These are still to be finished before your head... never behind the neck. Likewise, in the event that you are somebody who can as of now complete 3 arrangements of 6-8 force-ups, then you want to add weight. Search around online for what's known as a "pull-up belt" (likewise called a "plunge belt") and get one. It will permit you to add extra weight to body weight practices like force-ups and plunges. As long as you are doing this and are gradually progressing in some way over time, the progressive overload principle will be in effect and the results you want will follow.

MAINTAINING MUSCLE MASS

The human body has a normally happening measure still up in the air by hereditary qualities, sex-based chemicals, and age. You can prepare your body to build how much muscle by doing proactive tasks that invigorate muscle development and by consuming a bigger number of calories than you consume to help new tissue.

In any case, when you gain new muscle tissue, you can lose it because of done being animated or on the other hand assuming you eat less calories than you consume. The inborn bulk you have in your young adulthood will likewise decline as you age. Keeping up with muscle as you age is crucial for remaining free and practical in later life.

Step-by-step instructions to Keep up with Muscle Mass
There are a few stages you can take to keep up with your bulk and forestall muscle misfortune. Exercise and diet are both significant.

Work out with loads consistently.
Eat a lot of protein.
Consume an adequate number of calories.

Consolidate cardio and opposition preparing.

Get sufficient rest and rest.

Weight Train forever

From around the age of 30, we begin to lose muscle mass normally leisurely. This age-related muscle misfortune, known as sarcopenia, increments and turns out to be more evident after age 40, with a 30 to half downfall by age 80.

Purposes behind this muscle misfortune are blended, and the rate it happens for you relies upon a few hereditary and way of life factors. A decrease in sex chemicals and lower active work levels in maturing people are the essential culprits.

You can forestall, or if nothing else slow, this regular condition of misfortune by remaining dynamic. Work out with loads a few times every week, practicing all your significant muscle gatherings. Permit two days between exercises if conceivable.

Center around Protein

Guaranteeing that you eat well and get the suggested measure of protein for your action level will assist with keeping up with muscle as you age. You want somewhere around 0.8 grams of protein per kilogram of body weight day to day, and up to 1.2 grams is better for the individuals who are maturing and expecting to keep up with muscle mass.

To sort out how much protein you really want, take your weight in pounds, and duplicate it by 0.45. Duplicate that number by 1.2 to get your suggested everyday protein admission (in grams).

Protein is expected to assemble and keep up with muscle since it is answerable for tissue development and fix. Various examinations show that high protein admission is indispensable for safeguarding bulk as you age and when you are eating fewer carbs beneath upkeep calories.

More established people frequently undereat protein and can wind up putting themselves at a higher gamble of lack of protein. Different elements incorporate the conceivable diminished retention of protein as you age because of diminished stomach capability and bacteria.

In the event that you struggle with meeting your protein needs, consider adding protein powder to help your admission. Research recommends that older people can significantly profit from protein supplementation to guarantee they get to the point of supporting muscle maintenance.

Get An adequate number of Calories
Assume you don't eat (and drink) adequately to keep up with your body weight offset with how much energy you use in everyday living, including active work. All things considered, you will lose muscle and likely bone. Focusing on the general calories you consume can assist you with keeping up with your muscle.

While eating adequate protein is fundamental, and weighty mentors like competitors could require somewhat more protein than those referenced above, it is presumably much more basic to eat an adequate number of generally calories. Starches are fundamental for giving an anabolic (muscle building) boost in the body. In the event that you don't get enough, you could lose muscle.8

It is likewise fundamental to Refuel after work out. Taking in a few protein and sugars in no less than an hour of your exercise and adequately past that to refuel will assist with guaranteeing muscle upkeep and even development as you get an insulin spike.

In the event that you're a competitor, you really want to decide an optimal load for your action, keep a watch on the scales, and change your eating regimen and exercise as needs be. Profoundly dynamic individuals will require considerably more calories than the people who are inactive.

 What Happens When You Don't Eat Subsequent to Working Out?
Train to Help Muscle
The kind of preparation you do likewise assumes a part in muscle upkeep. As examined above, weight-bearing activity is imperative. While phenomenal for general well-being and sickness counteraction, cardiovascular activity won't go as far in safeguarding your muscle mass.

As a matter of fact, an excess of perseverance exercise can prompt muscle misfortune as the body endeavors to become lighter and more productive to fulfill needs. Notwithstanding, adding opposition preparing to your cardio workout daily practice as well as the other way around can work on your capacity to keep up with muscle.
The sort of opposition preparing you in all actuality do matters also. Zeroing in on hypertrophy style preparing, which is the sort that assists work with muscling mass, likewise forestalls muscle misfortune, regardless of whether you are in a calorie deficiency.

Lifting loads at least three times each week and preparing each body part no less than two times every week is ideal. You'll have to add volume and dynamically over-burden your muscles to keep seeing development or keep up with muscle.

 Activities to Forestall Muscle Misfortune

Unwind and Rest Enough
Rest is a period of modifying. Chemicals like testosterone and human development chemicals set about modifying and fixing your body. Relaxing rest assists with this interaction, so ensure you get it. Unwinding is significant too since close-to-home pressure will instigate catabolic

pressure chemicals, and that implies more obliteration of muscle on the off chance that you're not careful.12
Also, rest gives sufficient energy to your exercises and energizes better eating decisions. Additionally, recuperation time is vital for appropriate muscle development and upkeep.

In working out and powerlifting, individuals who don't normally convey or effectively improve muscle are frequently called "hard gainers." This sounds a little overly critical, yet it's more an assertion of truth. Individuals with an incline instead of a strong regular form are sorted deductively as ectomorphs.

The more ripped constructs are mesomorphs. Those that convey more fat normally may be endomorphs. Yet, don't overreact, there are many in the middle between, and you are not bound to an existence of a thin ectomorph.

CONCLUSION

No matter how much muscle mass you gain so far never forget it can still lessen and consistency is the only way to get it back on track. Eat healthy and properly to avoid losing muscle growth.

Several factors decide the amount of muscle you possess and how rapidly and how much you lose it as you age. Nonetheless, there are ways you can bring down the dangers of muscle misfortune by zeroing in on your eating routine, exercise, and way of life propensities.

 Muscle is fundamental for maturing in a functioning, autonomous, and sound way. Your possibilities of an excellent life and agony-free maturing are greatly improved assuming that you safeguard muscle

Focus on your diet and nutrition to keep your body in a more stabilized mode and with proper weight lifting and exercise you are good to go in gaining that muscle mass efficiently.

ABOUT THE AUTHOR

Personal trainer and bodybuilder, Williams Scott is a fitness expert in Los Angeles, California. His passion for fitness has not only been transformed into a thriving business but also into a book. In 2014, he published his first book, a set of workouts for beginning bodybuilders. The book's title is "Barbarian Warrior Workouts".

Williams Scott was inspired to write this book after realizing how many aspiring bodybuilders lacked proper guidance to build their body from a good beginning. He wanted to provide aspiring bodybuilders with information on how to bulk up and build muscle without straining their joints or joints. His advice is ideal for everyone, regardless of age, gender, or fitness level.